Mediterranean Diet Salad and Veggies Cookbook

50 healthy and nutritious salad and vegetable recipes to lose weight

Andrea Boni

Table of Contents

Introduction

Quick and straightforward Mediterranean diet recipes are all about vibrant vegetables and fruits cooked in one pot. All recipes are adorned with flavorful and tasty ingredients and in the end, garnish the dish with fresh coriander, fresh basil, and fresh parsley leaves.

What is the Mediterranean diet?

Welcome to the Mediterranean – a land of food, sunshine, rich culture, and a good lifestyle. The countries included in the Mediterranean – Italy, Greece, Turkey, Morocco, Libya, Egypt, Spain, and France. Following the Mediterranean diet – you will enjoy delicious and fresh food and health benefits. To summarize the Mediterranean diet:

- Eat fresh vegetable and fruit
- Nuts and olive oil
- Healthy Salad

Ingredients used in Mediterranean Diet

The Mediterranean diet is famous for its spices and ingredients. Each region has its specialties.

Olive oil:

Olive oil is the main ingredient used in these recipes. There are many health benefits of olive oil. Olive oil prevents heart diseases. The Mediterranean land is rich in olive trees.

Onion:

Other main ingredients used in these recipes are onions. Onions are an inexpensive ingredient and easy to find in any market. But, we recommend yellow onion for cooking and sweet onion for salad recipes. There are many health benefits of onions.

Garlic:

Garlic is mostly used in Mediterranean diet dishes. It is the most powerful ingredient – reduce blood pressure, protect from cancer, and control cholesterol.

Herbs:

Fresh or dried herbs are essential for Mediterranean diet dishes. Fresh parsley leaves used in salad or fresh mint leaves are also used in salad recipes. Many other herbs are used in the Mediterranean diet – oregano, thyme, basil, Marjoram, and Italian seasoning.

Cucumber Chicken Salad with Spicy Peanut Dressing

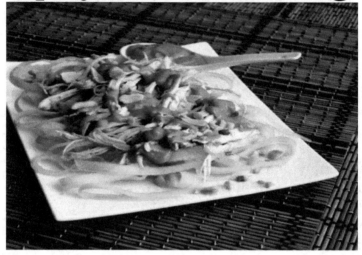

Cucumber chicken salad is a refreshing and healthy dish. It is dressed with peanuts. Yummy and mouthwatering dish served in lunch!

Preparation Time: 15 minutes
Cooking Time: 0 minutes
Servings: 2
Difficulty Level: Average

Ingredients:

- 1/2 cup peanut butter
- 1 tablespoon sambal oelek (chili paste)
- 1 tablespoon low-sodium soy sauce
- 1 teaspoon grilled sesame oil
- 4 tablespoons of water, or more if necessary
- 1 cucumber with peeled and cut into thin strips
- 1 cooked chicken fillet, grated into thin strips
- 2 tablespoons chopped peanuts

Directions:

Combine peanut butter, soy sauce, sesame oil, sambal oelek, and water in a bowl. Place the cucumber slices on a dish. Garnish with grated chicken and sprinkle with sauce. Sprinkle the chopped peanuts.

Nutrition (for100g):

720 calories 54g fat 8.9g carbohydrates 45.9g protein
733mg sodium

German Hot Potato Salad

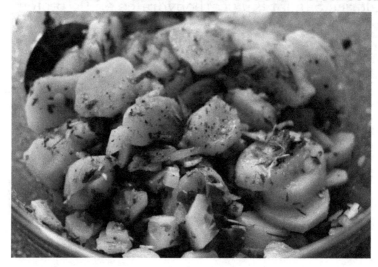

German potato salad is stuffed with peeled potatoes, celery seeds, white sugar, and slices of bacon. Serve it with lunch!

Preparation Time: 10 minutes
Cooking Time: 30 minutes
Servings: 12
Difficulty Level: Average

Ingredients:

- 9 peeled potatoes
- 6 slices of bacon
- 1/8 teaspoon ground black pepper
- 1/2 teaspoon celery seed
- 2 tablespoons white sugar
- 2 teaspoons salt
- 3/4 cup water
- 1/3 cup distilled white vinegar
- 2 tablespoons all-purpose flour
- 3/4 cup chopped onions

Directions:

Boil salted water in a large pot. Put in the potatoes and cook until soft but still firm, about 30 minutes. Drain, let cool and cut finely. Over medium heat, cook bacon in a pan. Drain, crumble and set aside. Save the cooking juices. Cook onions in bacon grease until golden brown.

Combine flour, sugar, salt, celery seed, and pepper in a small bowl. Add sautéed onions and cook, stirring until bubbling, and remove from heat. Stir in the water and vinegar, then bring back to the fire and bring to a boil, stirring constantly. Boil and stir. Slowly add bacon and potato slices to the vinegar/water mixture, stirring gently until the potatoes are warmed up.

Nutrition (for 100g):

205 calories 6.5g fat 32.9g carbohydrates 4.3g protein 814mg sodium

Chicken Fiesta Salad

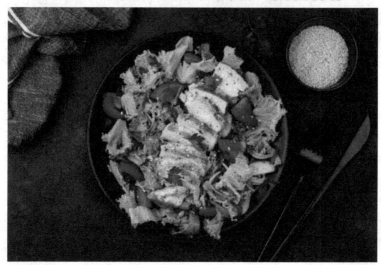

This dish is an attractive and creative – it is stuffed with green salad, Fajita, vegetable oil, chicken fillets, drained black beans, and tomatoes make it yummy dish.

Preparation Time: 20 minutes
Cooking Time: 20minutes
Servings: 4
Difficulty Level: Easy

Ingredients:

- 2 halves of chicken fillet without skin or bones
- 1 packet of herbs for fajitas, divided
- 1 tablespoon vegetable oil
- 1 can black beans, rinsed and drained
- 1 box of Mexican-style corn
- 1/2 cup of salsa
- 1 packet of green salad
- 1 onion, minced
- tomato, quartered

Directions:

Rub the chicken evenly with 1/2 of the herbs for fajitas. Cook the oil in a frying pan over medium heat and cook the chicken for 8 minutes on the side by side or until the juice is clear; put aside. Combine beans, corn, salsa, and other 1/2 fajita spices in a large pan. Heat over medium heat until lukewarm. Prepare the salad by mixing green vegetables, onion, and tomato. Cover the chicken salad and dress the beans and corn mixture.

Nutrition (for 100g):

311 calories 6.4g fat 42.2g carbohydrates 23g protein 853mg sodium

Corn & Black Bean Salad

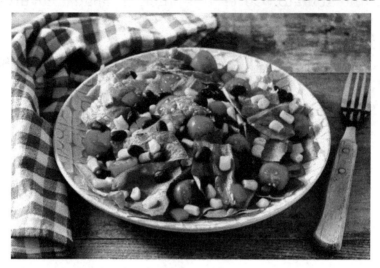

Black beans and corn salad is a refreshing and healthy dish. It is easy and quick side dish for any meal.

Preparation Time: 10 minutes
Cooking Time: 0 minutes
Servings: 4
Difficulty Level: Easy

Ingredients:

- tablespoons vegetable oil
- 1/4 cup balsamic vinegar
- 1/2 teaspoon of salt
- 1/2 teaspoon of white sugar
- 1/2 teaspoon ground cumin
- 1/2 teaspoon ground black pepper
- 1/2 teaspoon chili powder
- tablespoons chopped fresh coriander
- 1 can black beans (15 oz)
- 1 can of sweetened corn (8.75 oz) drained

Directions:

Combine balsamic vinegar, oil, salt, sugar, black pepper, cumin and chili powder in a small bowl. Combine black corn and beans in a medium bowl. Mix with vinegar and oil vinaigrette and garnish with coriander. Cover and refrigerate

overnight.
Nutrition (for 100g):
214 calories 8.4 g fat 28.6g carbohydrates 7.5g protein
415mg sodium

Awesome Pasta Salad

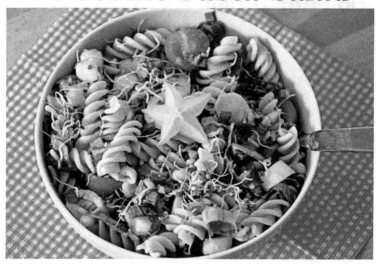

Pasta salad is a tasty and easy recipe. It is perfect side dish. This dish is blended with cherry tomatoes, fusilli pasta, sausage, and provolone cheese.

Preparation Time: 30 minutes
Cooking Time: 10 minutes
Servings: 16
Difficulty Level: Average

Ingredients:

- 1 (16-oz) fusilli pasta package
- 3 cups of cherry tomatoes
- 1/2 pound of provolone, diced
- 1/2 pound of sausage, diced
- 1/4 pound of pepperoni, cut in half
- 1 large green pepper
- 1 can of black olives, drained
- 1 jar of chilis, drained
- 1 bottle (8 oz) Italian vinaigrette

Directions:

Boil a lightly salted water in a pot. Stir in the pasta and cook for about 8 to 10 minutes or until al dente. Drain and rinse with cold water.

Combine pasta with tomatoes, cheese, salami, pepperoni, green pepper, olives, and peppers in a large bowl. Pour the vinaigrette and mix well.

Nutrition (for 100g):

310 calories 17.7g fat 25.9g carbohydrates 12.9g protein
746mg sodium

Tuna Salad

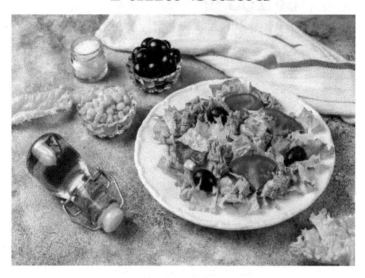

Tuna salad is a best version of salad. It is stuffed with garbanzo beans, mayonnaise, brown mustard, and tuna and make it yummy and spicy dish.

Preparation Time: 20 minutes
Cooking Time: 0 minutes
Servings: 4
Difficulty Level: Easy

Ingredients:
- (19 ounce) can of garbanzo beans
- 2 tablespoons mayonnaise
- teaspoons of spicy brown mustard
- tablespoon sweet pickle Salt and pepper to taste
- chopped green onions

Directions:
Combine green beans, mayonnaise, mustard, sauce, chopped green onions, salt and pepper in a medium bowl. Mix well.

Nutrition (for 100g):
220 calories 7.2g fat 32.7g carbohydrates 7g protein 478mg sodium

Southern Potato Salad

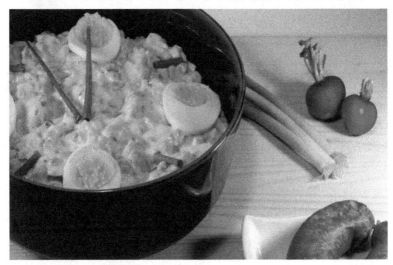

Potato salad is a light and fluffy meal. Learn how to make this tasty potato salad. It is ready in fifteen minutes.

Preparation Time: 15 minutes
Cooking Time: 15minutes
Servings: 4
Difficulty Level: Average

Ingredients:

- 4 potatoes
- 4 eggs
- 1/2 stalk of celery, finely chopped
- 1/4 cup sweet taste
- 1 clove of garlic minced
- 2 tablespoons mustard
- 1/2 cup mayonnaise
- salt and pepper to taste

Directions:

Boil water in a pot then situate the potatoes and cook until soft but still firm, about 15 minutes; drain and chop. Transfer the eggs in a pan and cover with cold water.

Boil the water; cover, remove from heat, and let the eggs soak in hot water for 10 minutes. Remove then shell and chop.

Combine potatoes, eggs, celery, sweet sauce, garlic, mustard, mayonnaise, salt, and pepper in a large bowl. Mix and serve hot.

Nutrition (for 100g):

460 calories 27.4g fat 44.6g carbohydrates 11.3g protein 214mg sodium

Seven-Layer Salad

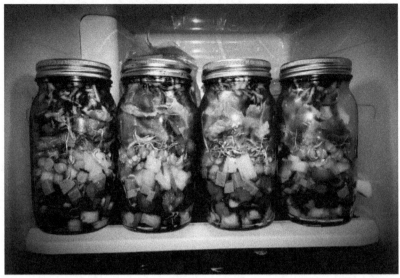

This bright, crunchy, and colorful seven-layer salad is full of flavor and yummy side dish. It is simple to prepare and ready in five minutes only!

Preparation Time: 15 minutes
Cooking Time: 5 minutes
Servings: 10
Difficulty Level: Average

Ingredients:

- 1-pound bacon
- 1 head iceberg lettuce
- 1 red onion, minced
- 1 pack of 10 frozen peas, thawed
- 10 oz grated cheddar cheese
- cup chopped cauliflower
- 1 1/4 cup mayonnaise
- tablespoons white sugar
- 2/3 cup grated Parmesan cheese

Directions:

Put the bacon in a huge, shallow frying pan. Bake over medium heat until smooth. Crumble and set aside. Situate the chopped lettuce in a large bowl and cover with a layer of an onion, peas, grated cheese, cauliflower, and bacon.

Prepare the vinaigrette by mixing the mayonnaise, sugar, and parmesan cheese. Pour over the salad and cool to cool.

Nutrition (for 100g):

387 calories 32.7g fat 9.9g carbohydrates 14.5g protein 609mg sodium

Kale, Quinoa &Avocado Salad with Lemon Dijon Vinaigrette

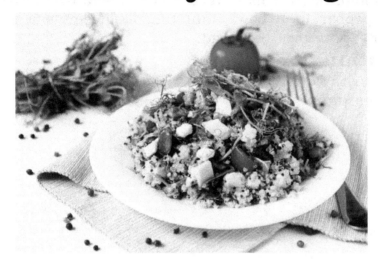

The combination of kale, quinoa, and avocado salad is tasty and healthy dish. Dressed with Dijon and lemon!

Preparation Time: 5 minutes
Cooking Time: 25 minutes
Servings: 4
Difficulty Level: Difficult

Ingredients:

- 2/3 cup of quinoa
- 1 1/3 cup of water
- bunch of kale, torn into bite-sized pieces
- 1/2 avocado - peeled, diced and pitted
- 1/2 cup chopped cucumber
- 1/3 cup chopped red pepper
- tablespoons chopped red onion
- 1 tablespoon of feta crumbled

Directions:

Boil the quinoa and 1 1/3 cup of water in a pan. Adjust heat and simmer until quinoa is tender and water is absorbed for about 15 to 20 minutes. Set aside to cool.

Place the cabbage in a steam basket over more than an inch of boiling water in a pan. Seal the pan with a lid and steam until hot, about 45 seconds; transfer to a large plate. Garnish with cabbage, quinoa, avocado, cucumber, pepper, red onion, and feta cheese.

Combine olive oil, lemon juice, Dijon mustard, sea salt, and black pepper in a bowl until the oil is emulsified in the dressing; pour over the salad.

Nutrition (for 100g):

342 calories 20.3g fat 35.4g carbohydrates 8.9g protein 705mg sodium

Chicken Salad

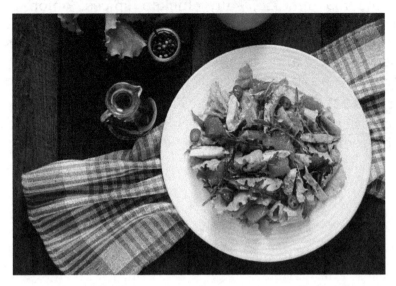

Chicken salad is undoubtedly a traditional recipe. Diced chicken is tossed with Swiss cheese, mayonnaise, green grapes, and aromatic spices.

Preparation Time: 20 minutes
Cooking Time: 0 minutes
Servings: 9
Difficulty Level: Easy

Ingredients:

- 1/2 cup mayonnaise
- 1/2 teaspoon of salt
- 3/4 teaspoon of poultry herbs
- 1 tablespoon lemon juice cups cooked chicken breast, diced
- 1/4 teaspoon ground black pepper
- 1/4 teaspoon garlic powder
- 1/4 teaspoon onion powder
- 1/2 cup finely chopped celery
- 1 (8 oz) box of water chestnuts, drained and chopped
- 1/2 cup chopped green onions
- 1 1/2 cups green grapes cut in half
- 1 1/2 cups diced Swiss cheese

Directions:

Combine mayonnaise, salt, chicken spices, onion powder, garlic powder, pepper, and lemon juice in a medium bowl. Combine chicken, celery, green onions, water chestnuts, Swiss cheese, and raisins in a big bowl. Stir in the mayonnaise mixture and coat. Cool until ready to serve.

Nutrition (for 100g):

293 calories 19.5g fat 1O.3g carbohydrates 19.4g protein 454mg sodium

Cobb Salad

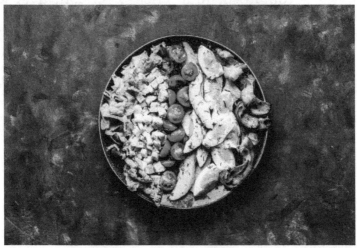

Cobb salad is stuffed with bacon slices, lettuce, and avocado. It is prepared in twenty minutes only. It is refreshing and mouthwatering dish.

Preparation Time: 5 minutes
Cooking Time: 15minutes
Servings: 6
Difficulty Level: Difficult

Ingredients:

- 6 slices of bacon
- 3 eggs
- 1 cup Iceberg lettuce, grated
- 3 cups cooked minced chicken meat
- 2 tomatoes, seeded and minced
- 3/4 cup of blue cheese, crumbled
- 1 avocado - peeled, pitted and diced
- 3 green onions, minced
- 1 bottle (8 oz.) Ranch Vinaigrette

Directions:

Situate the eggs in a pan and soak them completely with cold water. Boil the water. Cover and remove from heat and let the eggs rest in hot water for 1O to 12 minutes. Remove from hot water, let cool, peel, and chop. Situate the bacon in a big, deep frying pan. Bake over medium heat until smooth. Set aside.

Divide the grated lettuce into separate plates. Spread chicken, eggs, tomatoes, blue cheese, bacon, avocado, and green onions in rows on lettuce. Sprinkle with your favorite vinaigrette and enjoy.

Nutrition (for 100g):

525 calories 39.9g fat 1O.2g carbohydrates 31.7g protein 7O1mg sodium

Broccoli Salad

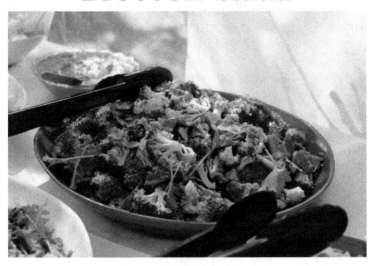

Broccoli is a healthy vegetable –there are many health benefits of this vegetable. Broccoli salad is a refreshing and nutrition salad recipe.

Preparation Time: 1O minutes
Cooking Time: 15minutes
Servings: 6
Difficulty Level: Average

Ingredients:

- 1O slices of bacon
- 1 cup fresh broccoli
- ¼ cup red onion, minced
- ½ cup raisins
  3 tablespoons white wine vinegar
- 2 tablespoons white sugar
- 1 cup mayonnaise
- cup of sunflower seeds

Directions:

Cook the bacon in a deep-frying pan over medium heat. Drain, crumble, and set aside. Combine broccoli, onion, and raisins in a medium bowl. Mix vinegar, sugar, and mayonnaise in a small bowl. Pour over the broccoli mixture and mix. Cool for at least two hours.

Before serving, mix the salad with crumbled bacon and

sunflower seeds.

Nutrition (for 100g):

559 calories 48.1g fat 31g carbohydrates 18g protein 584mg sodium

Strawberry Spinach Salad

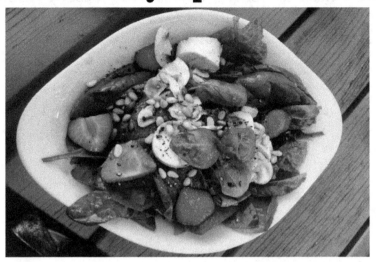

The combination of strawberry and spinach is crunchy and stunning. It is bright and colorful salad dish.

Preparation Time: 10 minutes
Cooking Time: 0 minutes
Servings: 4
Difficulty Level: Easy

Ingredients:
- tablespoons sesame seeds
- 1 tablespoon poppy seeds
- 1/2 cup white sugar
- 1/2 cup olive oil
- 1/4 cup distilled white vinegar
- 1/4 teaspoon paprika
- 1/4 teaspoon Worcestershire sauce
- 1 tablespoon minced onion
- 10 ounces fresh spinach
- 1-quart strawberries - cleaned, hulled and sliced
- 1/4 cup almonds, blanched and slivered

Directions:
In a medium bowl, whisk together the same seeds, poppy seeds, sugar, olive oil, vinegar, paprika, Worcestershire sauce, and onion. Cover, and chill for one hour.

In a large bowl, incorporate the spinach, strawberries, and almonds. Drizzle dressing over salad and toss. Refrigerate 10 to 15 minutes before serving.

Nutrition (for 100g):

491 calories 35.2g fat 42.9g carbohydrates 6g protein 691mg sodium

Pear Salad with Roquefort Cheese

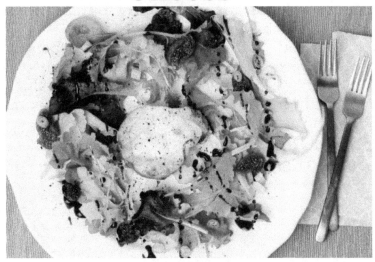

Pear salad is a yummy and mouthwatering dish recipe. It is stuffed with cheese, prepared mustard, and other flavorful ingredients.

Preparation Time: 20 minutes
Cooking Time: 10 minutes
Servings: 2
Difficulty Level: Average

Ingredients:

- 1 leaf lettuce, torn into bite-sized pieces
- 3 pears - peeled, cored and diced
- 5 ounces Roquefort, crumbled
- 1 avocado - peeled, seeded and diced
- 1/2 cup chopped green onions
- 1/4 cup white sugar
- 1/2 cup pecan nuts
- 1/3 cup olive oil
- 3 tablespoons red wine vinegar
- 1 1/2 teaspoon of white sugar
- 1 1/2 teaspoon of prepared mustard
- 1/2 teaspoon of salted black pepper
- 1 clove of garlic

Directions:

Stir in 1/4 cup of sugar with the pecans in a pan over medium heat. Continue to stir gently until the sugar caramelized with pecans. Cautiously transfer the nuts to wax paper. Let it chill and break into pieces.

Mix for vinaigrette oil, marinade, 1 1/2 teaspoon of sugar, mustard, chopped garlic, salt, and pepper.

In a deep bowl, combine lettuce, pears, blue cheese, avocado, and green onions. Put vinaigrette over salad, sprinkle with pecans and serve.

Nutrition (for 100g):

426 calories 31.6g fat 33.1g carbohydrates 8g protein 481mg sodium

Mexican Bean Salad

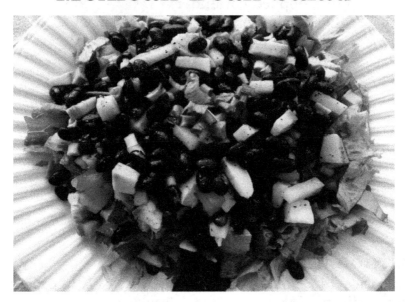

A colorful and spicy bean salad is a healthy and nourishing recipe. These are stuffed with black beans, red beans, white beans, and flavorful spices.

Preparation Time: 15 minutes
Cooking Time: 0 minutes
Servings: 6
Difficulty Level: Easy

Ingredients:

- 1 can black beans (15 oz), drained
- 1 can red beans (15 oz), drained
- 1 can white beans (15 oz), drained
- 1 green pepper, minced
- 1 red pepper, minced
- pack of frozen corn kernels
- 1 red onion, minced
- tablespoons fresh lime juice
- 1/2 cup olive oil
- 1/2 cup red wine vinegar
- 1 tablespoon lemon juice
- 1 tablespoon salt
- 2 tablespoons white sugar

- 1 clove of crushed garlic
- 1/4 cup chopped coriander
- 1/2 tablespoon ground cumin
- 1/2 tablespoon ground black pepper
- 1 dash of hot pepper sauce
- 1/2 teaspoon chili powder

Directions:

Combine beans, peppers, frozen corn, and red onion in a large bowl. Combine olive oil, lime juice, red wine vinegar, lemon juice, sugar, salt, garlic, coriander, cumin, and black pepper in a small bowl — season with hot sauce and chili powder.

Pour the vinaigrette with olive oil over the vegetables; mix well. Cool well and serve cold.

Nutrition (for 100g):

334 calories 14.8g fat 41.7g carbohydrates 11.2g protein 581mg sodium

Melon Salad

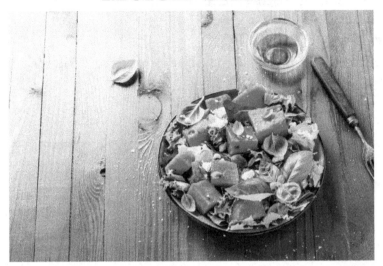

Melon salad is best dish for summer picnic. It will lose your weight and keeps you healthy. It needs simple ingredients.

Preparation Time: 20 minutes
Cooking Time: 0 minutes
Servings: 6
Difficulty Level: Average

Ingredients:

- ¼ teaspoon sea salt
- ¼ teaspoon black pepper
- 1 tablespoon balsamic vinegar
- cantaloupe, quartered &seeded
- 12 watermelon, small & seedless
- 2 cups mozzarella balls, fresh
- 1/3 cup basil, fresh & torn
- tbsp. olive oil

Directions:

Scrape out balls of cantaloupe, and the place them in a colander over a serving bowl. Use your melon baller to cut the watermelon as well, and then put them in with your cantaloupe.

Allow your fruit to drain for ten minutes, and then refrigerate the juice for another recipe. It can even be added to smoothies. Wipe the bowl dry, and then place your fruit in it.

Add in your basil, oil, vinegar, mozzarella and tomatoes before seasoning with salt and pepper. Gently mix and serve immediately or chilled.

Nutrition (for100g):

218 Calories13g Fat 9g Carbohydrates 1Og Protein 581mg Sodium

Orange Celery Salad

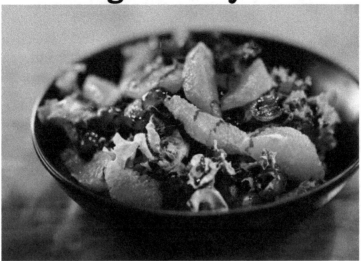

Orange and celery salad is a bright and juicy recipe. It is incredible and colorful salad dish. Top with sliced orange.

Preparation Time: 15 minutes
Cooking Time: O minutes
Servings: 6
Difficulty Level: Easy

Ingredients:
- tablespoon lemon juice, fresh
- ¼ teaspoon sea salt, fine
- ¼ teaspoon black pepper
- 1 tablespoon olive brine
- 1 tablespoon olive oil
- ¼ cup red onion, sliced
- ½ cup green olives
- oranges, peeled & sliced
- celery stalks, sliced diagonally in ½ inch slices

Directions:
Put your oranges, olives, onion and celery in a shallow bowl. In a different bowl whisk your oil, olive brine and lemon juice, pour this over your salad. Season with salt and pepper before serving.

Nutrition (for 100g):

65 Calories 7g Fats 9g Carbohydrates 2g Protein 614mg Sodium

Roasted Broccoli Salad

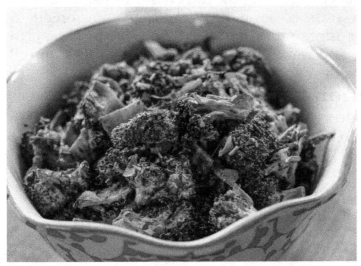

Roasted broccoli salad is a healthy and tasty dish. It has raw honey, balsamic vinegar, black pepper, bread cubes, and cherry tomatoes! It's yummy!

Preparation Time: 20 minutes
Cooking Time: 10minutes
Servings: 4
Difficulty Level: Difficult

Ingredients:
- 1 lb. broccoli, cut into florets & stem sliced
- 3 tablespoons olive oil, divided
- 1-pint cherry tomatoes
- 1 ½ teaspoons honey, raw & divided
- 3 cups cubed bread, whole grain
- 1 tablespoon balsamic vinegar
- ½ teaspoon black pepper
- ¼ teaspoon sea salt, fine grated parmesan for serving

Directions:
Prepare oven at 450 degrees, and then get outarimmed baking sheet. Place it in the oven to heat up. Drizzle your broccoli with a tablespoon of oil, and toss to coat.

Remove the baking sheet form the oven, and spoon the broccoli on it. Leave oil it eh bottom of the bowl, add in your tomatoes, toss to coat, and then toss your tomatoes with a tablespoon of honey. Pour them on the same baking sheet as your broccoli. Roast for fifteen minutes, and stir halfway through your cooking time. Add in your bread, and then roast for three more minutes. Whisk two tablespoons of oil, vinegar, and remaining honey. Season with salt and pepper. Pour this over your broccoli mix to serve.

Nutrition (for 100g):

226 Calories 12g Fat 26g Carbohydrates 7g Protein 581mg Sodium

Tomato Salad

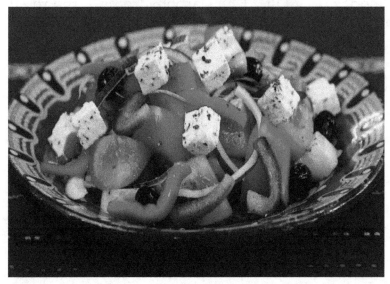

Tomato salad is a versatile and easy to prepare. This recipe is stuffed with cubes tomatoes, dried tomatoes, and season with sea salt and black pepper.

Preparation Time: 20 minutes
Cooking Time: 0 minutes
Servings: 4
Difficulty Level: Easy

Ingredients:
- 1 cucumber, sliced
- ¼ cup sun dried tomatoes, chopped
- 1 lb. tomatoes, cubed
- ½ cup black olives
- 1 red onion, sliced
- 1 tablespoon balsamic vinegar
- ¼ cup parsley, fresh & chopped
- 2 tablespoons olive oil
- sea salt & black pepper to taste

Directions:
Get out a bowl and combine all of your vegetables together. To make your dressing mix all your seasoning, olive oil and vinegar. Toss with your salad and serve fresh.

Nutrition (for 100g):

126 Calories 9.2g Fat 11.5g Carbohydrates 2.1g Protein
681mg Sodium

Feta Beet Salad

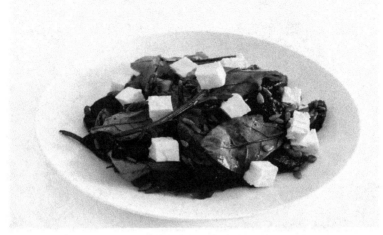

Beetroot is a healthy vegetable and the salad of this vegetable is awesome. It is tossed with olive oil.

Preparation Time: 15 minutes
Cooking Time: 0 minutes
Servings: 4
Difficulty Level: Easy

Ingredients:

- 6 red beets, cooked &peeled
- 3 ounces feta cheese, cubed
- 2 tablespoons olive oil
- 2 tablespoons balsamic vinegar

Directions:

- Combine everything together, and then serve.

Nutrition (for 100g):

230 Calories 12g Fat 26.3g Carbohydrates 7.3g Protein 614mg Sodium

Cauliflower &Tomato Salad

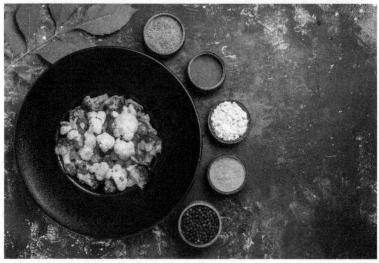

Cauliflower and tomato salad is a healthy and tasty recipe. It is ready in no minutes. It is good for summer picnic.

Preparation Time: 15 minutes
Cooking Time: 0 minutes
Servings: 4
Difficulty Level: Easy

Ingredients:

- head cauliflower, chopped
- tablespoons parsley, fresh chopped
- 2 cups cherry tomatoes, halved
- 2 tablespoons lemon juice, fresh
- 2 tablespoons pine nuts sea salt & black pepper to taste

Directions:

Mix your lemon juice, cherry tomatoes, cauliflower and parsley together, and then season. Top with pine nuts, and mix well before serving.

Nutrition (for 100g):

64 Calories 3.3g Fat 7.9g Carbohydrates 2.8g Protein 614mg Sodium

Pilaf with Cream Cheese

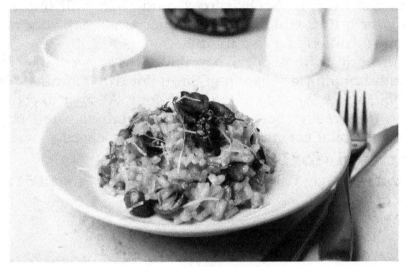

Pilaf with cream cheese has yellow grain rice, vegetable broth, and cayenne pepper and serves it in lunch!

Preparation Time: 20 minutes
Cooking Time: 10 minutes
Servings: 6
Difficulty Level: Average

Ingredients:

- 2 cups yellow long grain rice, parboiled
- 1 cup onion
- 4 green onions
- 3 tablespoons butter
- 3 tablespoons vegetable broth
- 2 teaspoons cayenne pepper
- 1 teaspoon paprika
- ½ teaspoon cloves, minced
- 2 tablespoons mint leaves, fresh & chopped
- 1 bunch fresh mint leaves to garnish
- 1 tablespoons olive oil
- sea salt & black pepper to taste

Cheese Cream:

- 3 tablespoons olive oil
- sea salt & black pepper to taste
- 9 ounces cream cheese

Directions:

Ready the oven at 360 degrees, and then pull out a pan. Heat your butter and olive oil together, and cook your onions and spring onions for two minutes.

Add in your salt, pepper, paprika, cloves, vegetable broth, rice and remaining seasoning. Sauté for three minutes. Wrap with foil, and bake for another half hour. Allow it to cool.

Mix in the cream cheese, cheese, olive oil, salt and pepper. Serve your pilaf garnished with fresh mint leaves.

Nutrition (for 100g):

364 Calories 30g Fat 20g Carbohydrates 5g Protein 511mg Sodium

Roasted Eggplant Salad

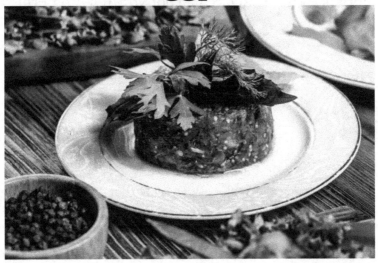

Eggplant is a healthy vegetable. Eggplant salad is stuffed with cherry tomatoes, oregano, and other flavorful ingredients.

Preparation Time: 10 minutes
Cooking Time: 20 minutes
Servings: 6
Difficulty Level: Easy

Ingredients:

- red onion, sliced
- tablespoons parsley, fresh &chopped
- 1 teaspoon thyme
- cups cherry tomatoes, halved sea salt & black pepper to taste
- 1 teaspoon oregano
- tablespoons olive oil
- 1 teaspoon basil
- 3 eggplants, peeled & cubed

Directions:

Start by heating your oven to 350. Season your eggplant with basil, salt, pepper, oregano, thyme and olive oil. Situate it on a baking tray, and bake for a half hour. Toss with your remaining ingredients before serving.

Nutrition (for 100g):

148 Calories 7.7g Fat 20.5g Carbohydrates 3.5g Protein
660mg Sodium

Roasted Veggies

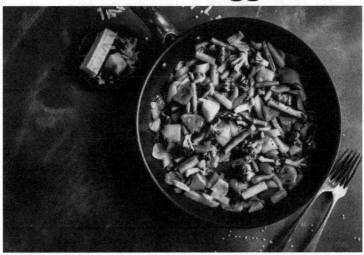

Roasted vegetable is another versatile dish. It is stuffed with zucchini, red bell pepper, rosemary, and tossed with olive oil.

Preparation Time: 5 minutes
Cooking Time: 15minutes
Servings: 12
Difficulty Level: Easy

Ingredients:

- 6 cloves garlic
- 6 tablespoons olive oil
- 1 fennel bulb, diced
- zucchini, diced
- red bell peppers, diced
- 6 potatoes, large &diced
- 2 teaspoons sea salt
- ½ cup balsamic vinegar
- ¼ cup rosemary, chopped & fresh
- 2 teaspoons vegetable bouillon powder

Directions:

Start by heating your oven to 400. Put your potatoes, fennel, zucchini, garlic and fennel on a baking dish, drizzling with olive oil. Sprinkle with salt, bouillon powder, and rosemary. Mix well, and then bake at 450 for thirty to forty minutes. Mix your vinegar into the vegetables before serving.

Nutrition (for 100g):

675 Calories 21g Fat 112g Carbohydrates 13g Protein 718mg Sodium

Pistachio Arugula Salad

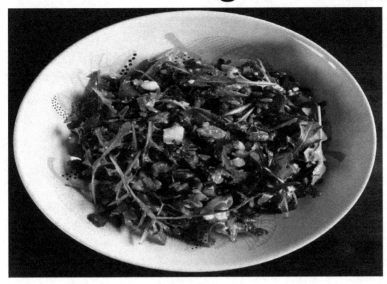

Arugula salad is a crunchy in each bite. The flavorful arugula salad is stuffed with pistachios and parmesan cheese.

Preparation Time: 20 minutes
Cooking Time: 0 minutes
Servings: 6
Difficulty Level: Easy

Ingredients:

- 6 cups kale, chopped
- ¼ cup olive oil
- 2 tablespoons lemon juice, fresh
- ½ teaspoon smoked paprika
- 2 cups arugula
- 1/3 cup pistachios, unsalted & shelled
- 6 tablespoons parmesan cheese, grated

Directions:

Get out a salad bowl and combine your oil, lemon, smoked paprika and kale. Gently massage the leaves for half a minute. Your kale should be coated well. Gently mix your arugula and pistachios when ready to serve.

Nutrition (for 100g):

15O Calories 12g Fat 8g Carbohydrates 5g Protein 637mg Sodium

Parmesan Barley Risotto

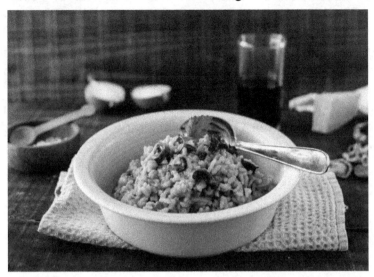

Barley is a rich and delicious dish – stuffed with cheese, white wine, and season with black pepper and salt.

Preparation Time: 10 minutes
Cooking Time: 20 minutes
Servings: 6
Difficulty Level: Difficult

Ingredients:

- 1 cup yellow onion, chopped
- 1 tablespoon olive oil
- 4 cups vegetable broth, low sodium
- 2 cups pearl barley, uncooked
- ½ cup dry white wine
- cup parmesan cheese, grated fine &divided sea salt & black pepper to taste
- fresh chives, chopped for serving lemon wedges for serving

Directions:

Add your broth into a saucepan and bring it to a simmer over medium-high heat. Get out a stock pot and put it over medium-high heat as well. Heat your oil before adding in your onion. Cook for eight minutes and stir occasionally. Add in your barley and cook for two minutes more. Stir in your barley, cooking until it's toasted.

Pour in the wine, cooking for a minute more. Most of the liquid should have evaporated before adding in a cup of warm broth. Cook and stir for two minutes. Your liquid should be absorbed. Add in the remaining broth by the cup, and cook until ach cup is absorbed. It should take about two minutes each time.

Pull out from the heat, add half a cup of cheese, and top with remaining cheese, chives, and lemon wedges.

Nutrition (for 100g):

345 Calories 7g Fat 56g Carbohydrates 14g Protein 912mg Sodium

Seafood &Avocado Salad

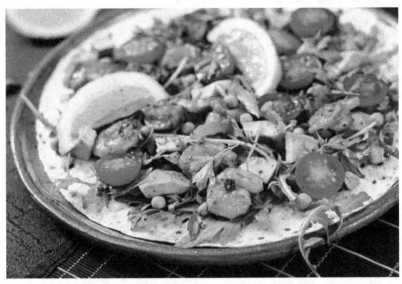

Seafood and avocado salad is a healthy and crunchy dish. The combination of shrimp and salmon is best. Top with mayonnaise.

Preparation Time: 10 minutes
Cooking Time: 0 minutes
Servings: 4
Difficulty Level: Easy

Ingredients:

- lbs. salmon, cooked &chopped
- 2 lbs. shrimp, cooked & chopped
- 1 cup avocado, chopped
- 1 cup mayonnaise
- 4 tablespoons lime juice, fresh
- 2 cloves garlic
- 1 cup sour cream
- sea salt & black pepper to taste
- ½ red onion, minced
- 1 cup cucumber, chopped

Directions:

Start by getting out a bowl and combine your garlic, salt, pepper, onion, mayonnaise, sour cream and lime juice,

Get out a different bowl and mix together your salmon, shrimp, cucumber, and avocado.

Add the mayonnaise mixture to your shrimp, and then allow it to sit for twenty minutes in the fridge before serving.

Nutrition (for 100g):

394 Calories 30g Fat 3g Carbohydrates 27g Protein 815mg Sodium

Mediterranean Shrimp Salad

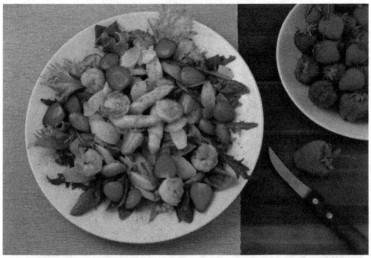

Shrimp salad is stuffed with celery stalk, mayonnaise, boiled egg, and green onions. Sprinkle with fresh parsley leaves.

Preparation Time: 40 minutes
Cooking Time: 0 minutes
Servings: 6
Difficulty Level: Easy

Ingredients:

- 1 ½ lbs. shrimp, cleaned & cooked
- 2 celery stalks, fresh onion
- green onions
- 4 eggs, boiled
- 3 potatoes, cooked
- 3 tablespoons mayonnaise
- sea salt & black pepper to taste

Directions:

Start by slicing your potatoes and chopping your celery. Slice your eggs, and season. Mix everything together. Put your shrimp over the eggs, and then serve with onion and green onions.

Nutrition (for100g):

207 Calories 6g Fat 15g Carbohydrates17g Protein 664mg Sodium

Chickpea Pasta Salad

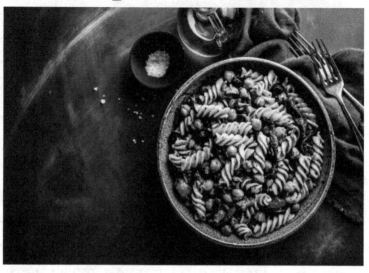

The gorgeous chickpeas salad is packed with fresh and minced oregano and parsley, and tossed with red wine.

Preparation Time: 10 minutes
Cooking Time: 15minutes
Servings: 6
Difficulty Level: Average

Ingredients:

- 2 tablespoons olive oil
- 16 ounces rotelle pasta
- ½ cup cured olives, chopped
- 2 tablespoons oregano, fresh & minced
- 2 tablespoons parsley, fresh &chopped
- 1 bunch green onions, chopped
- ¼ cup red wine vinegar
- 15 ounces canned garbanzo beans, drained & rinsed
- ½ cup parmesan cheese, grated sea salt & black pepper to taste

Directions:

Boil water and put the pasta al dente and follow per package instructions. Drain it and rinse it using cold water.
Get out a skillet and heat your olive oil over medium heat. Add in your scallions, chickpeas, parsley, oregano and

olives. Decrease the heat, and sauté for twenty minutes more. Allow this mixture to cool.

Toss your chickpea mixture with your pasta and add in your grated cheese, salt, pepper and vinegar. Let it chill for four hours or overnight before serving.

Nutrition (for 100g):

424 Calories 10g Fat 69g Carbohydrates 16g Protein 714mg Sodium

Mediterranean Stir Fry

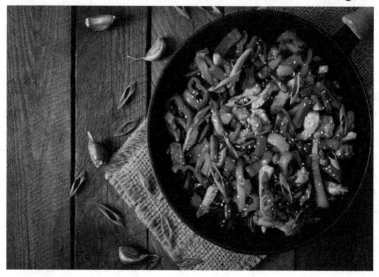

Mediterranean stir-fry recipe is stuffed with zucchini, chicken breast, red pepper flakes, and cooked barley. Top with fresh basil.

Preparation Time: 10 minutes
Cooking Time: 30 minutes
Servings: 4
Difficulty Level: Average

Ingredients:

- 1 onion
- ¼ teaspoon sea salt
- 2 cloves garlic
- 3 teaspoons olive oil, divided
- 1 lb. chicken breasts, boneless
- 1 cup quick cooking barley
- 2 cups water
- ¼ teaspoon black pepper
- 1 teaspoon oregano
- ¼ teaspoon red pepper flakes
- ½ teaspoon basil
- 2 plum tomatoes
- ½ cup Greek olives, pitted
- 1 tablespoons parsley, fresh

- 2 zucchinis

Directions:

Start by removing the skin from your chicken, and then chop it into smaller pieces. Chop the garlic and parsley, and then chop your olives, zucchini, tomatoes and onions. Get out a saucepan and bring your water to a boil.

Mix in your barley, letting it simmer for eight to ten minutes. Turn off heat. Let it rest for five minutes. Get out a skillet and add in two teaspoons of olive oil. Stir fry your chicken once it's hot, and then remove it from heat. Cook the onion in your remaining oil. Mix in your remaining ingredients, and cook for an additional three to five minutes. Serve warm.

Nutrition (for 100g):

337 Calories 8.6g Fat 32.3g Carbohydrates 31.7g Protein 517mg Sodium

Balsamic Cucumber Salad

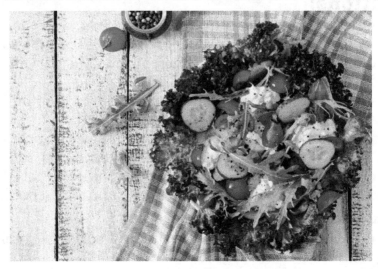

Cucumber is a healthy vegetable – it is stuffed with English cucumber, red onion, balsamic vinaigrette, and grape tomatoes. Top with feta cheese.

Preparation Time: 15 minutes
Cooking Time: 0 minutes
Servings: 4
Difficulty Level: Easy

Ingredients:

- 2/3 large English cucumber, halved and sliced
- 2/3 medium red onion, halved and thinly sliced
- 5 1/2 tablespoons balsamic vinaigrette
- 1/3 cups grape tomatoes, halved
- 1/2 cup crumbled reduced-fat feta cheese

Directions:

In a big bowl, mix cucumber, tomatoes and onion. Add vinaigrette; toss to coating. Refrigerate, covered, till serving. Just prior to serving, stir in cheese. Serve with a slotted teaspoon.

Nutrition (for 100g):

250 calories 12g fats 15g carbohydrates 34g protein 633mg Sodium

Beef Kefta Patties with Cucumber Salad

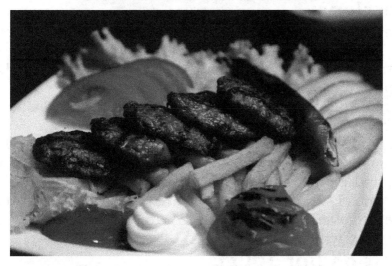

Beef kefta patties are tasty and wonderful salad recipe. Top with chopped fresh parsley and chopped fresh coriander. Serve with sauce.

Preparation Time: 10 minutes
Cooking Time: 15 minutes
Servings: 2
Difficulty Level: Difficult

Ingredients:

- cooking spray
- 1/2-pound ground sirloin
- tablespoons plus
- 2 tablespoons chopped fresh flat-leaf parsley, divided
- 1/2 teaspoons chopped peeled fresh ginger
- 1 teaspoon ground coriander
- tablespoons chopped fresh cilantro
- 1/4 teaspoon salt
- 1/2 teaspoon ground cumin
- 1/4 teaspoon ground cinnamon
- cup thinly sliced English cucumbers
- 1 tablespoon rice vinegar
- 1/4 cup plain fat-free Greek yogurt

- 1 1/2 teaspoons fresh lemon juice
- 1/4 teaspoon freshly ground black pepper
- 1 (6-inch) pitas, quartered

Directions:

Warmth a grill skillet over medium-high warmth. Coat pan with cooking spray. Combine beef, 1/4 glass parsley, cilantro, and next 5 elements in a medium bowl. Divide combination into 4 the same portions, shaping each into a 1/2-inch-thick patty. Add patties to pan; cook both sides until desired degree of doneness.

Mix cucumber and vinegar in a medium bowl; throw well. Combine fat-free yogurt, remaining 2 tablespoons parsley, juice, and pepper in a little bowl; stir with a whisk. Set up 1 patty and 1/2 cup cucumber mixture on each of 4 china. Top each offering with about 2 tablespoons yogurt spices. Serve each with 2 pita wedges.

Nutrition (for 100g):

116 calories 5g fats 11g carbohydrates 28g protein 642mg sodium

Chicken and Cucumber Salad with Parsley Pesto

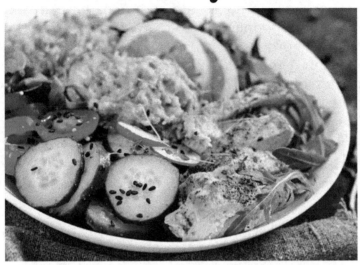

Chicken and cucumber salad is a fresh and tasty salad. Top with fresh parsley pesto. It is ready in five minutes.

Preparation Time: 15 minutes
Cooking Time: 5 minutes
Servings: 8
Difficulty Level: Easy

Ingredients:

- 2/3 cups packed fresh flat-leaf parsley leaves
- 1 1/3 cups fresh baby spinach
- 1 1/2 tablespoons toasted pine nuts
- 1 1/2 tablespoons grated Parmesan cheese
- 2 1/2 tablespoons fresh lemon juice
- 1 1/3 teaspoons kosher salt
- 1/3 teaspoon black pepper
- 1 1/3 medium garlic cloves, smashed
- 2/3 cup extra-virgin olive oil
- 5 1/3 cups shredded rotisserie chicken (from 1 chicken)
- 2 2/3 cups cooked shelled edamame
- 1 1/2 cans 1 (15-oz.) unsalted chickpeas, drained and rinsed

- 1 1/3 cups chopped English cucumbers
- 1/3 cups loosely packed arugula

Directions:

Combine parsley, spinach, lemon juice, pine nuts, cheese, garlic, salt, and pepper in food processor; process about 1 minute. With processor running, add oil; process until smooth, about 1 minute.

Stir together chicken, edamame, chickpeas, and cucumber in a large bowl. Add pesto; toss to combine.

Place 2/3 cup arugula in each of 6 bowls; top each with 1 cup chicken salad mixture. Serve immediately.

Nutrition (for 100g):

116 calories 12g fats 3g carbohydrates 9g protein 663mg sodium

Easy Arugula Salad

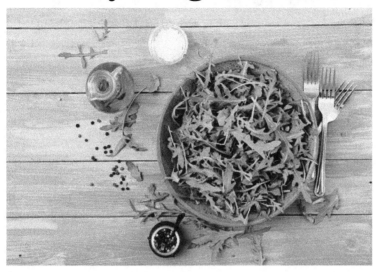

Each bite of arugula salad is crunchy and tasty. The combination of pine nuts, cherry tomatoes, and parmesan cheese is perfect.

Preparation Time: 15 minutes
Cooking Time: 0 minutes
Servings: 6
Difficulty Level: Easy

Ingredients:

- cups young arugula leaves, rinsed and dried
- 1 1/2 cups cherry tomatoes, halved
- 6 tablespoons pine nuts
- 3 tablespoons grape seed oil or olive oil
- 1 1/2 tablespoons rice vinegar
- 3/8 teaspoon freshly ground black pepper to taste
- 6 tablespoons grated Parmesan cheese
- 3/4 teaspoon salt to taste
- 1 1/2 large avocados - peeled, pitted and sliced

Directions:

In a sizable plastic dish with a cover, incorporate arugula, cherry tomatoes, pine nut products, oil, vinegar, and Parmesan cheese. Period with salt and pepper to flavor. Cover, and wring to mix.

Separate salad onto china, and top with slices of avocado.

Nutrition (for 100g):

120 calories 12g fats 14g carbohydrates 25g protein 736mg sodium

Feta Garbanzo Bean Salad

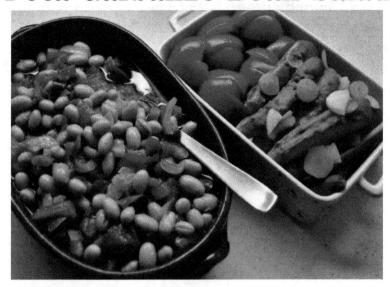

Garbanzo bean salad is loaded with olives, fresh parsley, English cucumber, sliced red onion and other flavorful ingredients.

Preparation Time: 10 minutes
Cooking Time: 0 minutes
Servings: 6
Difficulty Level: Easy

Ingredients:

- 1 1/2 cans (15 ounces) garbanzo beans
- 1 1/2 cans (2-1/4 ounces) sliced ripe olives, drained
- 1 1/2 medium tomatoes
- 6 tablespoons thinly sliced red onions
- 2 1/4 cups
- 1-1/2 coarsely chopped English cucumbers
- 6 tablespoons chopped fresh parsley
- 4 1/2 tablespoons olive oil
- 3/8 teaspoon salt
- 1 1/2 tablespoons lemon juice
- 3/16 teaspoon pepper
- 7 1/2 cups mixed salad greens
- 3/4 cup crumbled feta cheese

Directions:

Transfer all ingredients in a big bowl; toss to combine. Add parmesan cheese.

Nutrition (for100g):

140 calories16g fats10g carbohydrates 24g protein 817mg sodium

Greek Brown and Wild Rice Bowls

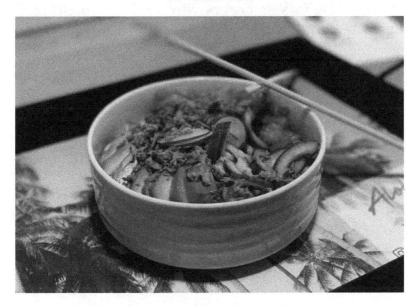

Greek brown rice is a yummy and tasty dish. Serve it with raita, green chutney, and chili-sauce.

Preparation Time: 15 minutes
Cooking Time: 5 minutes
Servings: 4
Difficulty Level: Easy

Ingredients:

- 2 packages (8-1/2 ounces) ready-to-serve whole grain brown and wild rice medley medium ripe avocado, peeled and sliced
- 1 1/2 cups cherry tomatoes, halved
- 1/2 cup Greek vinaigrette, divided
- 1/2 cup crumbled feta cheese
- 1/2 cup pitted Greek olives, sliced minced fresh parsley, optional

Directions:

Inside a microwave-safe dish, mix the grain mix and 2 tablespoons vinaigrette. Cover and cook on high until warmed through, about 2 minutes. Divide between 2 bowls.

Best with avocado, tomato vegetables, cheese, olives, leftover dressing and, if desired, parsley.

Nutrition (for 100g):

116 calories 10g fats 9g carbohydrates 26g protein 607mg sodium

Greek Dinner Salad

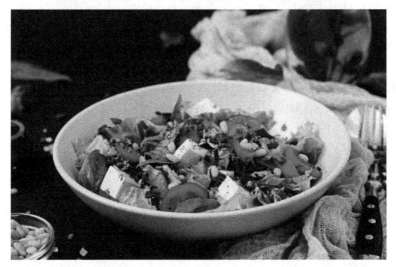

Greek salad is a tasty and healthy recipe. It is loaded with fresh parsley, chopped dill, Romaine lettuce, and cucumber and makes a yummy salad dish.

Preparation Time: 10 minutes
Cooking Time: 0 minutes
Servings: 4
Difficulty Level: Easy

Ingredients:

- 1/2 tablespoons coarsely chopped fresh parsley
- 2 tablespoons coarsely chopped fresh dill
- 2 teaspoons fresh lemon juice
- 2/3 teaspoon dried oregano
- 2 teaspoons extra virgin olive oil
- 4 cups shredded Romaine lettuce
- 2/3 cup thinly sliced red onions
- 1/2 cup crumbled feta cheese
- 2 cups diced tomatoes
- 2 teaspoons capers
- 2/3 cucumber, peeled, quartered lengthwise, and thinly sliced
- 2/3 (19-ounce) can chickpeas, drained and rinsed
- 4 (6-inch) whole wheat pitas, each cut into
- 8 wedges

Directions:

Combine the first 5 substances in a sizable dish; stir with a whisk. Add a member of the lettuce family and the next 6 ingredients (lettuce through chickpeas); throw well. Serve with pita wedges.

Nutrition (for100g):

103 calories12g fats 8g carbohydrates 36g protein 813mg sodium

Halibut with Lemon-Fennel Salad

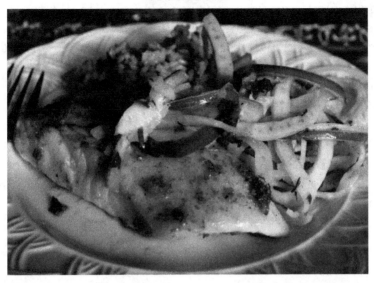

Halibut and fennel salad – it is stuffed with ground coriander, sliced onion, ground cumin, halibut, and lemon-fennel. Top with lemon wedge!

Preparation Time: 15 minutes
Cooking Time: 5 minutes
Servings: 2
Difficulty Level: Average

Ingredients:

- 1/2 teaspoon ground coriander
- 1/4 teaspoon salt
- 1/8 teaspoon freshly ground black pepper
- 2 1/2 teaspoons extra-virgin olive oils, divided
- 1/4 teaspoon ground cumin
- 1 garlic clove, minced
- 2 (6-ounce) halibut fillets
- 1 cup fennel bulb
- 2 tablespoons thinly vertically sliced red onions
- 1 tablespoon fresh lemon juice
- 1 1/2 teaspoons chopped flat-leaf parsley
- 1/2 teaspoon fresh thyme leaves

Directions:

Combine the first 4 substances in a little dish. Combine 1/2 tsp spice mixture, 2 teaspoons oil, and garlic in a little bowl; rub garlic clove mixture evenly over fish. Heat 1 teaspoon oil in a sizable nonstick frying pan over medium-high high temperature. Add fish to pan; cook 5 minutes on each side or until the desired level of doneness.

Combine remaining 3/4 teaspoon spice mix, remaining 2 tsp oil, fennel light bulb, and remaining substances in a medium bowl, tossing well to coat.

Provide salad with seafood.

Nutrition (for 100g):

11O calories 9g fats 11g carbohydrates 29g protein 558mg sodium

Herbed Greek Chicken Salad

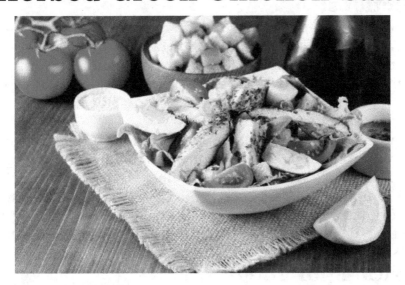

Greek chickpea is a tasty and delicious dish. It is a healthy and nutritious and stuffed with chicken breast and fat-free yogurt.

Preparation Time: 10 minutes
Cooking Time: 10 minutes
Servings: 2
Difficulty Level: Average

Ingredients:

- 1/2 teaspoon dried oregano
- 1/4 teaspoon garlic powder
- 3/8 teaspoon black pepper, divided cooking spray
- 1/2-pound skinless, boneless chicken breasts, cut into
- 1-inch cubes
- 1/4 teaspoon salt, divided
- 1/2 cup plain fat-free yogurt
- 1 teaspoon tahini (sesame-seed paste)
- 2 1/2 tsps. Fresh lemon juice
- 1/2 teaspoon bottled minced garlic
- 4 cups chopped Romaine lettuce
- 1/2 cup peeled chopped English cucumbers
- 1/2 cup grape tomatoes, halved
- 3 pitted kalamata olives, halved

- 2 tablespoons (1 ounce) crumbled feta cheese

Directions:

Combine oregano, garlic natural powder, 1/2 teaspoon pepper, and 1/4 tsp salt in a bowl. Heat a nonstick skillet over medium-high heat. Coating pan with cooking food spray. Add poultry and spice combination; sauté until poultry is done. Drizzle with 1 teaspoon juice; stir. Remove from pan.

Combine remaining 2 teaspoons juice, leftover 1/4 teaspoon sodium, remaining 1/4 tsp pepper, yogurt, tahini, and garlic in a little bowl; mix well. Combine member of the lettuce family, cucumber, tomatoes, and olives. Put 2 1/2 cups of lettuce mixture on each of 4 plates. Top each serving with 1/2 cup chicken combination and 1 teaspoon cheese. Drizzle each serving with 3 tablespoons yogurt combination

Nutrition (for 100g):

116 calories 11g fats 15g carbohydrates 28g protein 634mg sodium

Greek Couscous Salad

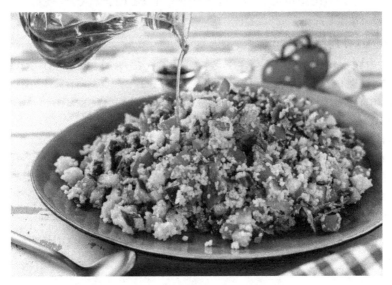

A delicious and healthy Greek salad is a yummy and mouthwatering dish. Tossed with olive oil and lemon zest!

Preparation Time: 10 minutes
Cooking Time: 15minutes
Servings: 10
Difficulty Level: Easy

Ingredients:

- 1 can (14-1/2 ounces) reduced-sodium chicken broth
- 1 1/2 cups
- 1-3/4 uncooked whole wheat couscous (about 11 ounces)

Dressing:

- 6 1/2 tablespoons olive oil
- 1 1/4 teaspoons
- 1-1/2 grated lemon zest
- 3 1/2 tablespoons lemon juice
- 13/16 teaspoon adobo seasonings
- 3/16 teaspoon salt

Salad:

- 1 2/3 cups grape tomatoes, halved
- 5/6 English cucumber, halved lengthwise and sliced
- 3/4 cup coarsely chopped fresh parsley

- 1 can (6-1/2 ounces) sliced ripe olives, drained
- 6 1/2 tablespoons crumbled feta cheese
- 3 1/3 green onions, chopped

Directions:

In a sizable saucepan, bring broth to a boil. Stir in couscous. Remove from heat; let stand, covered, until broth is absorbed, about 5 minutes. Transfer to a sizable dish; cool completely.

Beat together dressing substances. Add cucumber, tomato vegetables, parsley, olives and green onions to couscous; stir in dressing. Gently mix in cheese. Provide immediately or refrigerate and serve frosty.

Nutrition (for 100g):

114 calories 13g fats 18g carbohydrates 27g protein 811mg sodium

Barley Risotto with Tomatoes

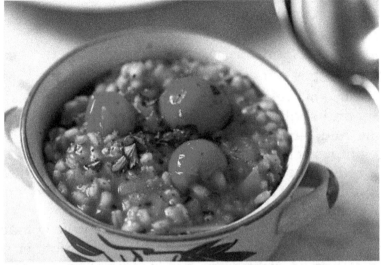

Barley ricotta tomatoes are stuffed with shallots, vegetable stock, smoked paprika, and other fresh and flavorful ingredients. Top with fresh parsley

Preparation Time: 20 minutes
Cooking Time: 45 minutes
Servings: 4
Difficulty Level: Average

Ingredients:

- 2 tablespoons extra-virgin olive oil
- 2 celery stalks, diced
- ½ cup shallots, diced
- 4 garlic cloves, minced
- 3 cups no-salt-added vegetable stock
- 1 (14.5-ounce) can no-salt-added diced tomatoes
- 1 (14.5-ounce) can no-salt-added crushed tomatoes
- 1 cup pearl barley
- Zest of 1 lemon
- 1 teaspoon kosher salt
- ½ teaspoon smoked paprika
- ¼ teaspoon red pepper flakes
- ¼ teaspoon freshly ground black pepper
- 4 thyme sprigs

- dried bay leaf
- cups baby spinach
- ½ cup crumbled feta cheese
- 1 tablespoon fresh oregano, chopped
- tablespoon fennel seeds, toasted (optional)

Directions:

Cook the olive oil in a large saucepan over medium heat. Add the celery and shallots and sauté, about 4 to 5 minutes. Add the garlic and sauté 30 seconds. Add the vegetable stock, diced tomatoes, crushed tomatoes, barley, lemon zest, salt, paprika, red pepper flakes, black pepper, thyme, and the bay leaf, and mix well. Let it boil, then lower to low, and simmer. Cook, stirring occasionally, for 40minutes.

Remove the bay leaf and thyme sprigs. Stir in the spinach. In a small bowl, combine the feta, oregano, and fennel seeds. Serve the barley risotto in bowls topped with the feta mixture.

Nutrition (for 100g):

375 Calories 12g Fat 13g Carbohydrates 11g Protein 799mg Sodium

Chickpeas and Kale with Spicy Pomodoro Sauce

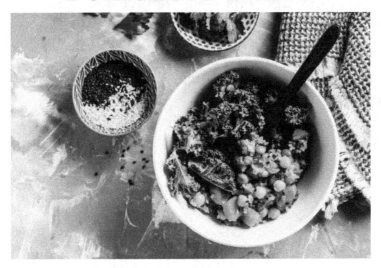

Chickpeas and kale bowl is a healthy and tasty dish. It is ready in thirty-five minutes with flavorful ingredients. Top with sliced tomatoes.

Preparation Time: 10 minutes
Cooking Time: 35 minutes
Servings: 4
Difficulty Level: Easy

Ingredients:

- tablespoons extra-virgin olive oil
- 4 garlic cloves, sliced
- 1 teaspoon red pepper flakes
- 1 (28-ounce) can no-salt-added crushed tomatoes
- 1 teaspoon kosher salt
- ½ teaspoon honey
- bunch kale, stemmed and chopped
- (15-ounce) cans low-sodium chickpeas, drained and rinsed
- ¼ cup fresh basil, chopped
- ¼ cup grated pecorino Romano cheese

Directions:

Cook the olive oil in a sauté pan over medium heat. Stir in the garlic and red pepper flakes and sauté until the garlic is a light golden brown, about 2 minutes. Add the tomatoes, salt, and honey and mix well. Reduce the heat to low and simmer for 20 minutes.

Add the kale and mix in well. Cook about 5 minutes. Add the chickpeas and simmer about 5 minutes. Remove from heat and stir in the basil. Serve topped with pecorino cheese.

Nutrition (for 100g):

420 Calories 13g Fat 12g Carbohydrates 20g Protein 882mg Sodium

Roasted Feta with Kale and Lemon Yogurt

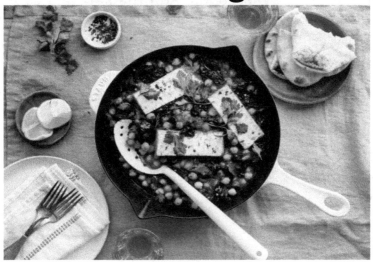

Roasted feta is stuffed with yummy and spicy ingredients. It is ready in twenty minutes. Top with feta cheese.

Preparation Time: 15 minutes
Cooking Time: 20 minutes
Servings: 4
Difficulty Level: Average

Ingredients:

- 1 tablespoon extra-virgin olive oil
- 1 onion, julienned
- ¼ teaspoon kosher salt
- 1 teaspoon ground turmeric
- ½ teaspoon ground cumin
- ½ teaspoon ground coriander
- ¼ teaspoon freshly ground black pepper
- 1 bunch kale, stemmed and chopped
- 7-ounce block feta cheese, cut into ¼-inch-thick slices
- ½ cup plain Greek yogurt
- 1 tablespoon lemon juice

Directions:

Preheat the oven to 400°F. Fry the olive oil in a large

ovenproof skillet or sauté pan over medium heat. Add the onion and salt; sauté until lightly golden brown, about 5 minutes. Add the turmeric, cumin, coriander, and black pepper; sauté for 30 seconds. Add the kale and sauté about 2 minutes. Add ½ cup water and continue to cook down the kale, about 3 minutes.

Remove from the heat and place the feta cheese slices on top of the kale mixture. Introduce in the oven and bake until the feta softens, 10 to 12 minutes. In a small bowl, combine the yogurt and lemon juice. Serve the kale and feta cheese topped with the lemon yogurt.

Nutrition (for 100g):

210 Calories 14g Fat 2g Carbohydrates 11g Protein 836mg Sodium

Roasted Eggplant and Chickpeas with Tomato Sauce

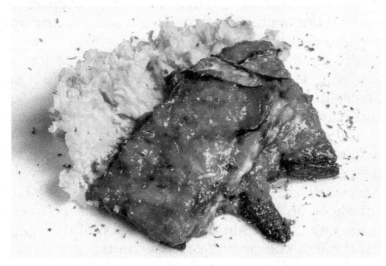

Roasted eggplant is stuffed with fresh oregano, feta cheese, crushed tomatoes, fresh basil, and tossed with olive oil.

Preparation Time: 15 minutes
Cooking Time: 60 minutes
Servings: 4
Difficulty Level: Difficult

Ingredients:

- Olive oil cooking spray
- 1 large (about 1 pound) eggplant, sliced into
- ¼-inch-thick rounds
- 1 teaspoon kosher salt, divided
- 1 tablespoon extra-virgin olive oil
- 3 garlic cloves, minced
- 1 (28-ounce) can no-salt-added crushed tomatoes
- ½ teaspoon honey
- ¼ teaspoon freshly ground black pepper
- 2 tablespoons fresh basil, chopped
- 1 (15-ounce) can no-salt-added or low-sodium chickpeas, drained and rinsed
- ¾ cup crumbled feta cheese
- 1 tablespoon fresh oregano, chopped

Directions:

Preheat the oven to 425°F. Grease and line two baking sheets with foil and lightly spray with olive oil cooking spray. Spread the eggplant in a single layer and sprinkle with ½ teaspoon of the salt. Bake for 20 minutes, turning once halfway, until lightly golden brown.

Meanwhile, heat the olive oil in a large saucepan over medium heat. Mix in the garlic and sauté for 30 seconds. Add the crushed tomatoes, honey, the remaining ½ teaspoon salt, and black pepper. Simmer about 20 minutes, until the sauce reduces a bit and thickens. Stir in the basil.

After removing the eggplant from the oven, reduce the oven temperature to 375°F. In a large rectangular or oval baking dish, spoon in the chickpeas and 1 cup sauce. Layer the eggplant slices on top, overlapping as necessary to cover the chickpeas. Lay the remaining sauce on top of the eggplant.

Sprinkle the feta cheese and oregano on top.

Wrap the baking dish with foil and bake for 15 minutes. Pull out the foil and bake an additional 15 minutes.

Nutrition (for 100g):

320 Calories 11g Fat 12g Carbohydrates 14g Protein 773mg Sodium

Baked Falafel Sliders

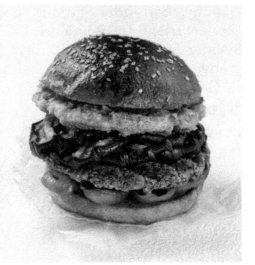

Falafel sliders are a yummy and delicious recipe. It is a healthy and mouthwatering recipe. Top with mayonnaise and tomato ketchup.

Preparation Time: 10 minutes
Cooking Time: 30 minutes
Servings: 6
Difficulty Level: Average

Ingredients:

- (15-ounce) can low-sodium chickpeas, drained and rinsed
- 1 onion, roughly chopped
- garlic cloves, peeled
- 2 tablespoons fresh parsley, chopped
- 2 tablespoons whole-wheat flour
- ½ teaspoon ground coriander
- ½ teaspoon ground cumin
- ½ teaspoon baking powder
- ½ teaspoon kosher salt
- ¼ teaspoon freshly ground black pepper
- Olive oil cooking spray

Directions:

Preheat the oven to 350°F. Put parchment paper or foil and

lightly spray with olive oil cooking spray in the baking sheet. In a food processor, mix in the chickpeas, onion, garlic, parsley, flour, coriander, cumin, baking powder, salt, and black pepper. Blend until smooth.

Make 6 slider patties, each with a heaping ¼ cup of mixture, and arrange on the prepared baking sheet. Bake for 30 minutes. Serve.

Nutrition (for 100g):

90 Calories 1g Fat 3g Carbohydrates 4g Protein 803mg Sodium

Portobello Caprese

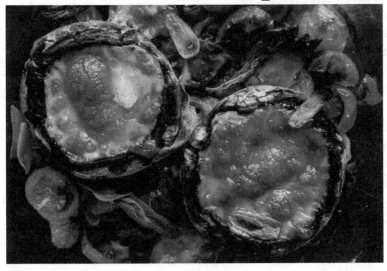

The caprese is a cheesy and delicious recipe. It is stuffed with cherry tomatoes, Portobello mushrooms, and mozzarella and parmesan cheese.

Preparation Time: 15 minutes
Cooking Time: 30minutes
Servings: 2
Difficulty Level: Difficult

Ingredients:

- 1 tablespoon olive oil
- 1 cup cherry tomatoes
- Salt and black pepper, to taste
- 4 large fresh basil leaves, thinly sliced, divided
- 3 medium garlic cloves, minced
- 2 large portobello mushrooms, stems removed
- 4 pieces mini Mozzarella balls
- 1 tablespoon Parmesan cheese, grated

Directions:

Prepare the oven to 350°F (180°C). Grease a baking pan with olive oil. Drizzle 1 tablespoon olive oil in a nonstick skillet, and heat over medium- high heat. Add the tomatoes to the skillet, and sprinkle salt and black pepper to season. Prick some holes on the tomatoes for juice during the cooking. Put the lid on and cook the tomatoes for 10 minutes or until tender.

Reserve 2 teaspoons of basil and add the remaining basil and garlic to the skillet. Crush the tomatoes with a spatula, then cook for half a minute. Stir constantly during the cooking. Set aside. Arrange the mushrooms in the baking pan, cap side down, and sprinkle with salt and black pepper totaste.

Spoon the tomato mixture and Mozzarella balls on the gill of the mushrooms, then scatter with Parmesan cheese to coat well. Bake until the mushrooms are fork-tender and the cheeses are browned. Pull out the stuffed mushrooms from the oven and serve with basil on top.

Nutrition (for 100g):

285 Calories 21.8g Fat 2.1g Carbohydrates 14.3g Protein 823mg Sodium

Mushroom and Cheese Stuffed Tomatoes

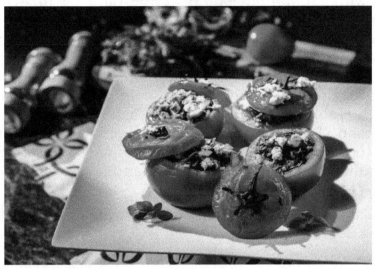

Stuffed tomatoes are loaded with cremini mushrooms, fresh basil, yellow onion, fresh oregano, and other flavorful ingredients.

Preparation Time: 15 minutes
Cooking Time: 20 minutes
Servings: 4
Difficulty Level: Average

Ingredients:

- 4 large ripe tomatoes
- 1 tablespoon olive oil
- ½ pound (454 g) white or cremini mushrooms, sliced
- 1 tablespoon fresh basil, chopped
- ½ cup yellow onion, diced
- 1 tablespoon fresh oregano, chopped
- 2 garlic cloves, minced
- ½ teaspoon salt
- ¼ teaspoon freshly ground black pepper
- 1 cup part-skim Mozzarella cheese, shredded
- 1 tablespoon Parmesan cheese, grated

Directions:

Ready the oven to 375°F (190°C). Cut a ½-inch slice off the top of each tomato. Scoop the pulp into a bowl and leave ½-inch tomato shells. Arrange the tomatoes on a baking sheet lined with aluminum foil. Heat the olive oil in a nonstick skillet over medium heat.

Add the mushrooms, basil, onion, oregano, garlic, salt, and black pepper to the skillet and sauté for 5 minutes.

Pour the mixture to the tomato pulp bowl, then add the Mozzarella cheese and stir to combine well. Spoon the mixture into each tomato shell, then top with a layer of Parmesan. Bake in the preheated oven for 15 minutes or until the cheese is bubbly and the tomatoes are soft. Pull out the stuffed tomatoes from the oven and serve warm.

Nutrition (for 100g):

254 Calories 14.7g Fat 5.2g Carbohydrates 17.5g Protein 783mg Sodium

Tabbouleh

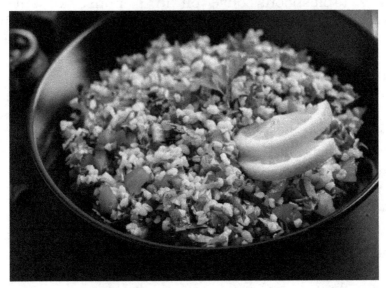

Learn how to prepare real Tabbouleh dish....! It is stuffed with riced cauliflower, cucumber, and season with black pepper and salt.

Preparation Time: 15 minutes
Cooking Time: 5minutes
Servings: 6
Difficulty Level: Average

Ingredients:

- 4 tablespoons olive oil, divided
- 4 cups riced cauliflower
- 3 garlic cloves, finely minced Salt and black pepper, to taste
- ½ large cucumber, peeled, seeded, and chopped
- ½ cup Italian parsley, chopped
- Juice of 1 lemon
- 2 tablespoons minced red onion
- ½ cup mint leaves, chopped
- ½ cup pitted Kalamata olives, chopped
- 1 cup cherry tomatoes, quartered
- 2 cups baby arugula or spinach leaves
- medium avocados, peeled, pitted, and diced

Directions:

Warm 2 tablespoons olive oil in a nonstick skillet over medium-high heat. Add the rice cauliflower, garlic, salt, and black pepper to the skillet and sauté for 3 minutes or until fragrant. Transfer them to a large bowl.

Add the cucumber, parsley, lemon juice, red onion, mint, olives, and remaining olive oil to the bowl. Toss to combine well. Reserve the bowl in the refrigerator for at least 30 minutes.

Remove the bowl from the refrigerator. Add the cherry tomatoes, arugula, and avocado to the bowl. Season well, and toss to combine well. Serve chilled.

Nutrition (for 100g):

198 Calories 17.5g Fat 6.2g Carbohydrates 4.2g Protein 773mg Sodium

Spicy Broccoli Rabe and Artichoke Hearts

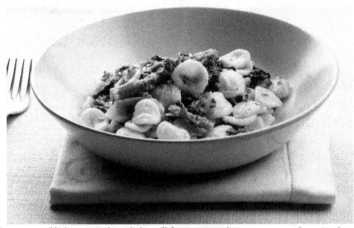

Spicy broccoli is cooked in fifteen minutes only. It is stuffed with fresh broccoli, red flakes pepper, artichokes, and season with pepper.

Preparation Time: 5 minutes
Cooking Time: 15 minutes
Servings: 4
Difficulty Level: Average

Ingredients:

- tablespoons olive oil, divided
- 2 pounds (907 g) fresh broccoli rabe
- 3 garlic cloves, finely minced
- 1 teaspoon red pepper flakes
- teaspoon salt, plus more to taste
- 13.5 ounces (383 g) artichoke hearts
- 1 tablespoon water
- tablespoons red wine vinegar
- Freshly ground black pepper, to taste

Directions:

Warm 2 tablespoons olive oil in a nonstick skillet over medium-high skillet. Add the broccoli, garlic, red pepper flakes, and salt to the skillet and sauté for 5 minutes or until the broccoli is soft.

Put the artichoke hearts to the skillet and sauté for 2 more minutes or until tender. Add water to the skillet and turn down the heat to low. Put the lid on and simmer for 5 minutes. Meanwhile, combine the vinegar and 1 tablespoon of olive oil in a bowl.

Drizzle the simmered broccoli and artichokes with oiled vinegar, and sprinkle with salt and black pepper. Toss to combine well before serving.

Nutrition (for 100g):

272 Calories 21.5g Fat 9.8g Carbohydrates 11.2g Protein 736mg Sodium

Shakshuka

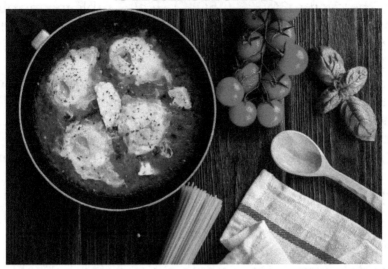

Shakshuka is an easy and delicious recipe – it is simple and healthy dish. Top with sliced yellow onions, smoked paprika, and chopped capers.

Preparation Time: 10 minutes
Cooking Time: 25minutes
Servings: 4
Difficulty Level: Difficult

Ingredients:

- 5 tablespoons olive oil, divided
- 1 red bell pepper, finely diced
- ½ small yellow onion, finely diced
- 14 ounces (397 g) crushed tomatoes, with juices
- 6 ounces (170 g) frozen spinach, thawed and drained of excess liquid
- teaspoon smoked paprika
- garlic cloves, finely minced
- 2 teaspoons red pepper flakes
- 1 tablespoon capers, roughly chopped
- 1 tablespoon water
- 6 large eggs
- ¼ teaspoon freshly ground black pepper
- ¾ cup feta or goat cheese, crumbled
- ¼ cup fresh flat-leaf parsley or cilantro, chopped

Directions:

Ready the oven to300°F (150°C).Heat 2 tablespoons olive oil in an oven- safe skillet over medium-high heat. Sauté the bell pepper and onion to the skillet until the onion is translucent and the bell pepper is soft.

Add the tomatoes and juices, spinach, paprika, garlic, red pepper flakes, capers, water, and 2 tablespoons olive oil to the skillet. Stir well and bring to a boil. Set down the heat to low, then put the lid on and simmer for 5 minutes.

Crack the eggs over the sauce, keep a little space between each egg, leave the egg intact and sprinkle with freshly ground black pepper. Cook until the eggs reach the right doneness.

Scatter the cheese over the eggs and sauce, and bake in the preheated oven for 5 minutes or until the cheese is frothy and golden brown. Drizzle with the remaining 1 tablespoon olive oil and spread the parsley on top before serving warm.

Nutrition (for 100g):

335 Calories 26.5g Fat 5g Carbohydrates 16.8g Protein 736mg Sodium

Conclusion

Thank you for pick-up for my *"Mediterranean diet salad and veggies cookbook."* 50-healthy and mouthwatering recipes will help you in weight loss.

CPSIA information can be obtained
at www.ICGtesting.com
Printed in the USA
LVHW081147240321
682294LV00007B/460

9 781801 797566